Dr. Seuss

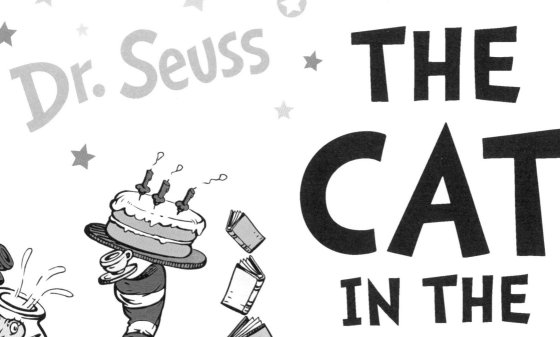

THE CAT IN THE HAT

Activity Book

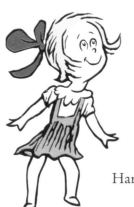

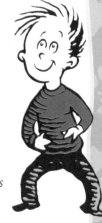

HarperCollins *Children's Books*

One rainy day

It's a rainy day and Sally and her brother are stuck indoors.
Let's connect the numbers to complete the picture!

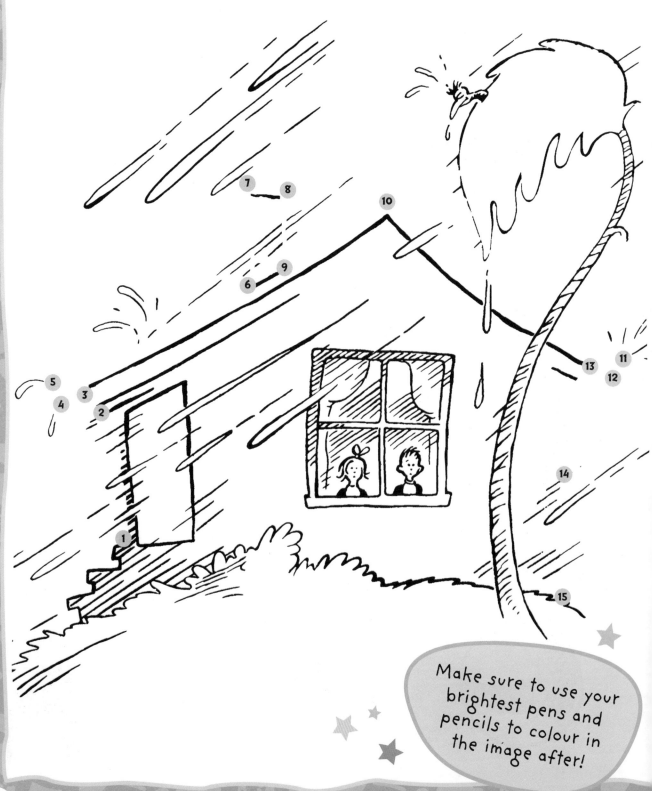

Make sure to use your brightest pens and pencils to colour in the image after!

Perfect pairs

Below are some of Sally and her brother's favourite toys!
Can you match up the pictures with their descriptions below?

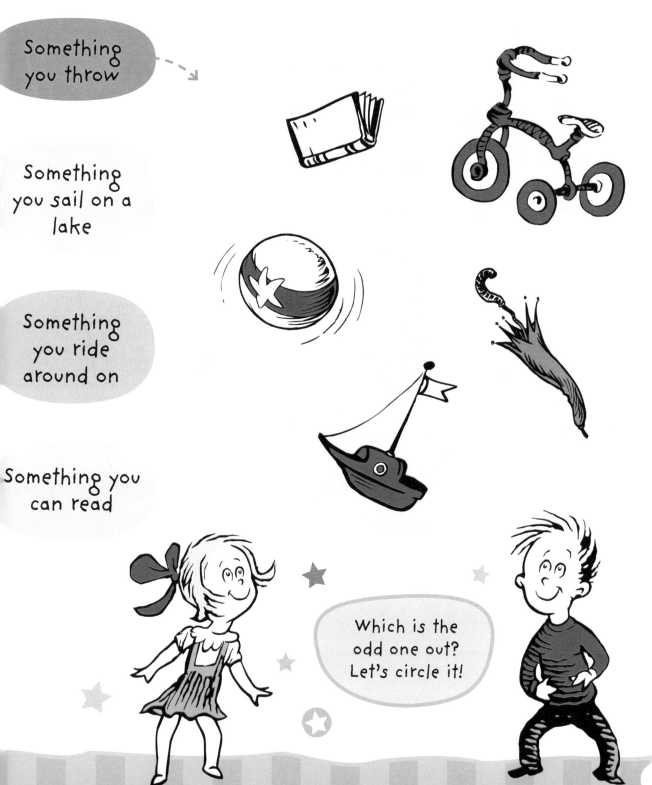

Something you throw

Something you sail on a lake

Something you ride around on

Something you can read

Which is the odd one out? Let's circle it!

An unexpected visitor

Find the stickers to match the colourful shadows here!

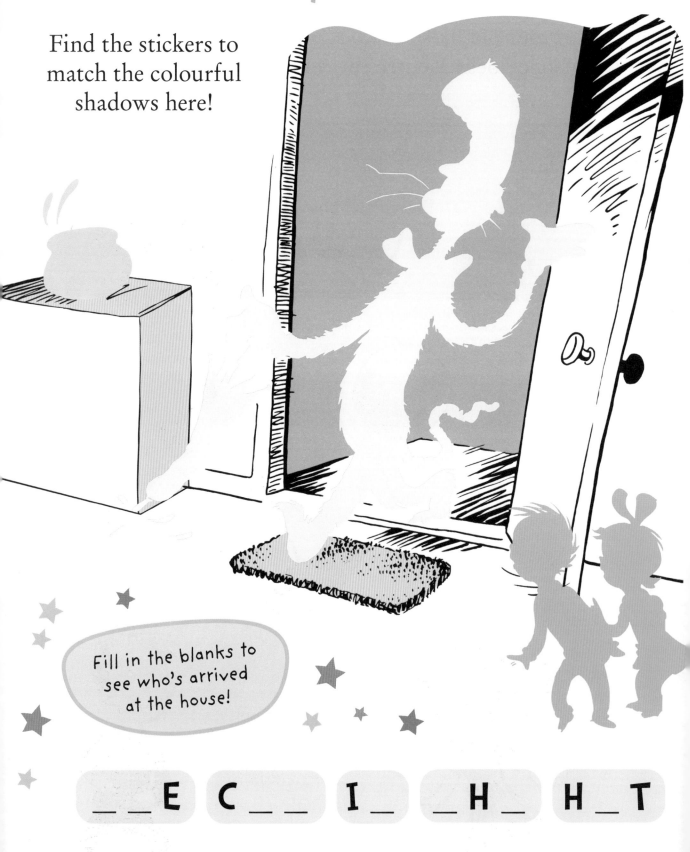

Fill in the blanks to see who's arrived at the house!

_ _ E C _ _ I _ _H_ H_T

One odd cat

Look at the four pictures below. Can you spot which one doesn't match the others?

Add a star sticker to the odd one out.

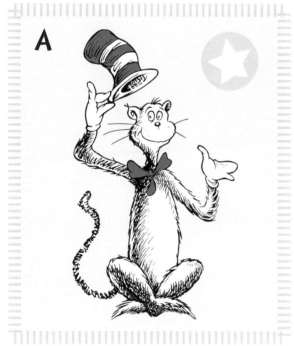

A

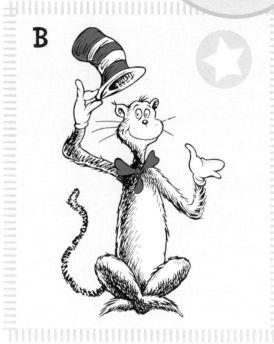

B

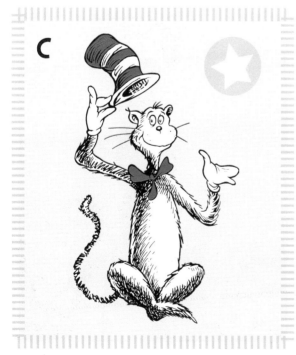

C

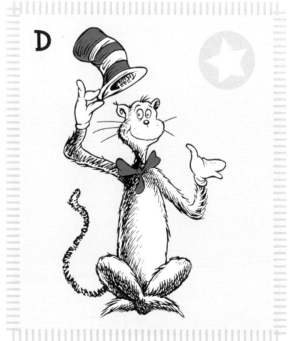

D

Super storytime

Let's find the matching stickers for the text below!

We 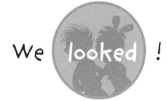 !

Then we saw him step in on the 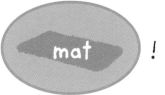 !

We looked!

And we saw him!

The 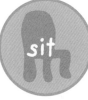 in the Hat!

And he said to us,

"Why do you there like that?"

"I know it is wet

And the 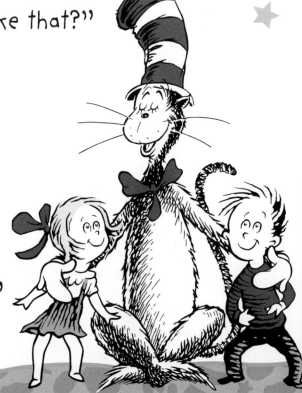 is not sunny.

But we can have

Lots of good fun that is funny!"

6

A balancing act

The Cat in the Hat is juggling!
How many things can you see in this picture?

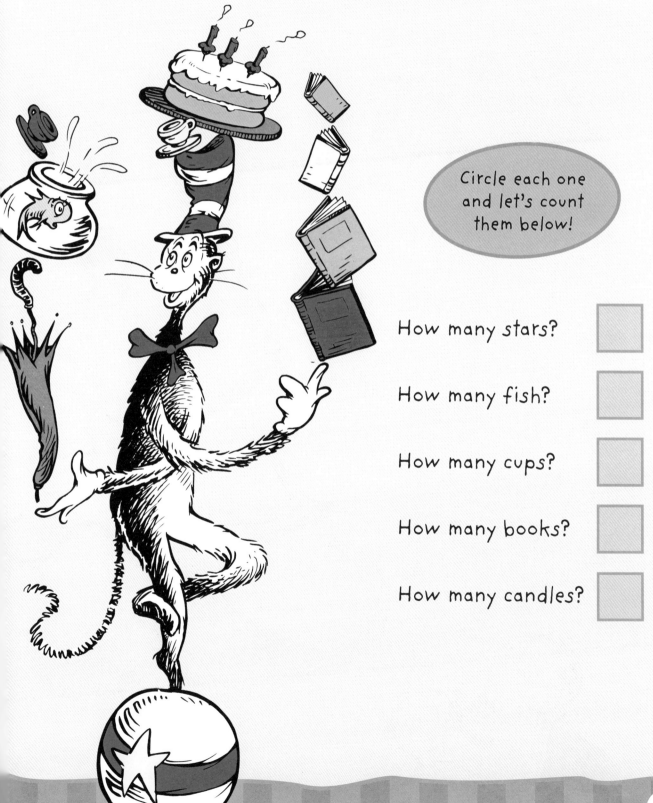

Circle each one and let's count them below!

How many stars? ☐

How many fish? ☐

How many cups? ☐

How many books? ☐

How many candles? ☐

A-maze-ing fun!

The Cat in the Hat is losing his balance! Can Sally and her brother get to the fish before he falls from the air?

Use your pen to draw a path to the fish — make sure you don't touch the edges!

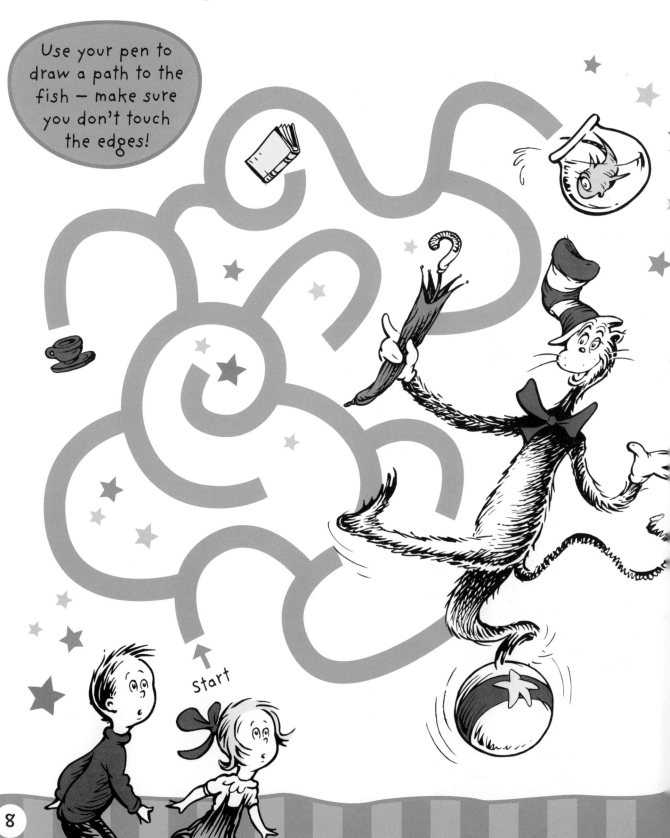

start

All fall down!

Down falls the Cat in the Hat! Use your best colours to fill in the picture below.

Be as imaginative and creative as you like!

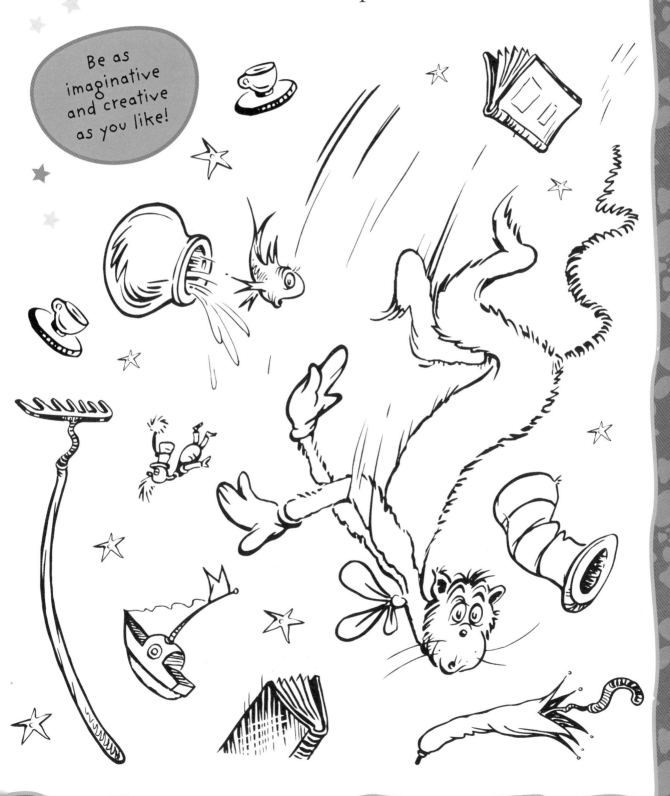

Puzzle pieces

What a mess! Use your stickers to complete the puzzle below.

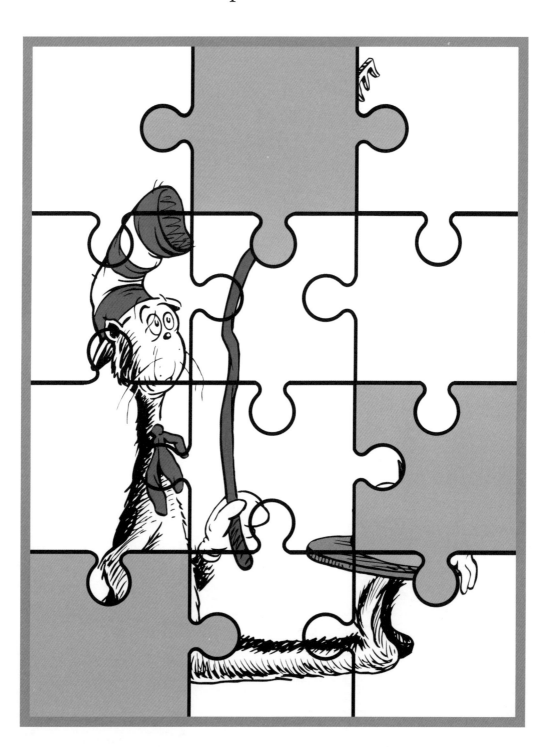

Fish frowns!

This fish does not look happy that the Cat in the Hat has come to play! Let's copy him on to the grid below.

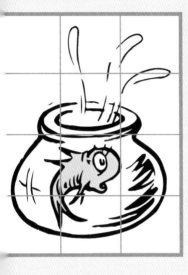

Colour in the fish once you've drawn him.

The Things' tracks

Trace the path to draw a line from Thing One to Thing Two.

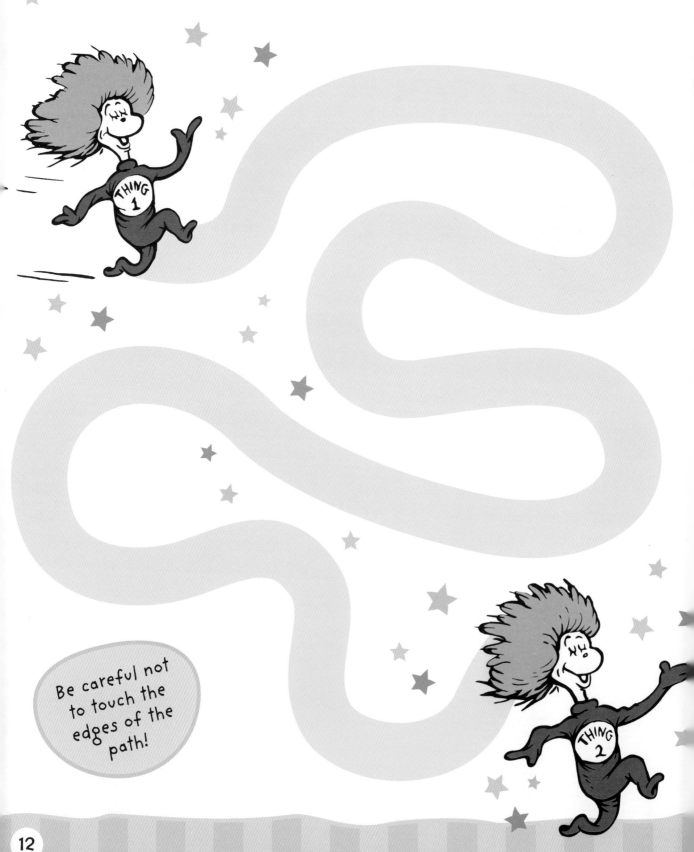

Be careful not to touch the edges of the path!

A new friend

Look at these four pictures below.
Which one doesn't match the others?

Add a star sticker to the odd one out.

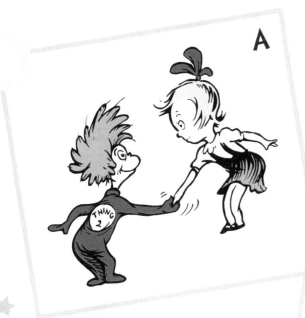

A

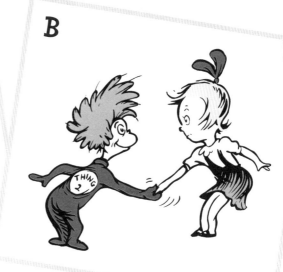

B

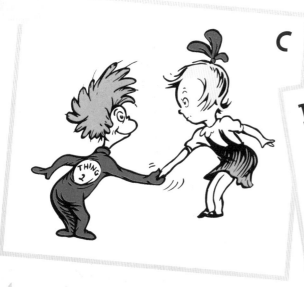

C

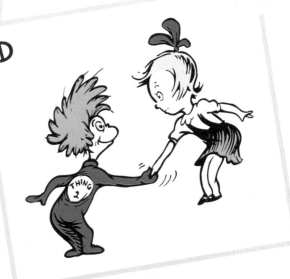

D

Cat-astrophic chaos!

The Cat in the Hat has released Thing One and Thing Two and they've turned the house upside down! Can you find and circle these parts of the bigger picture?

Add a star sticker when you've found each item.

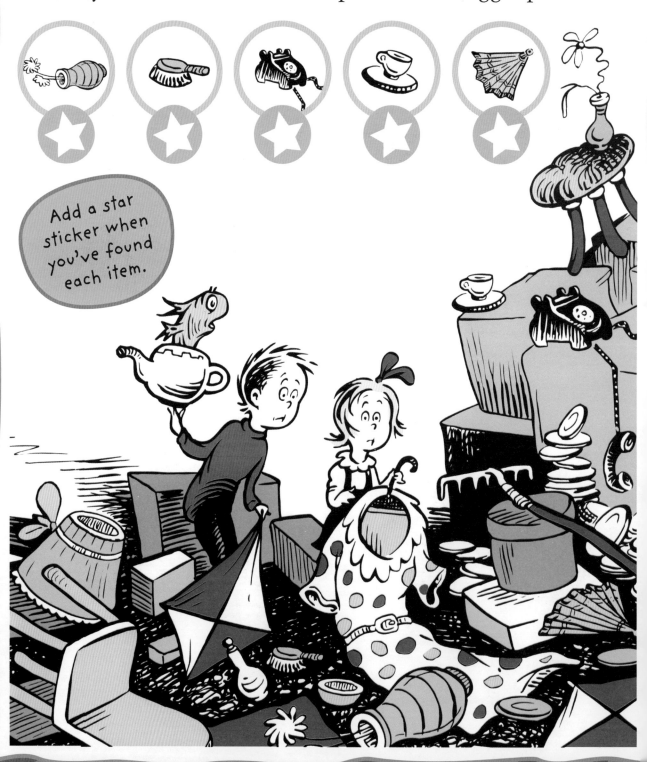

14

Maze muddle

Can you help Sally and her brother get from one side of the maze to the Cat in the Hat?

Start →

Count the fish you pass on your way.

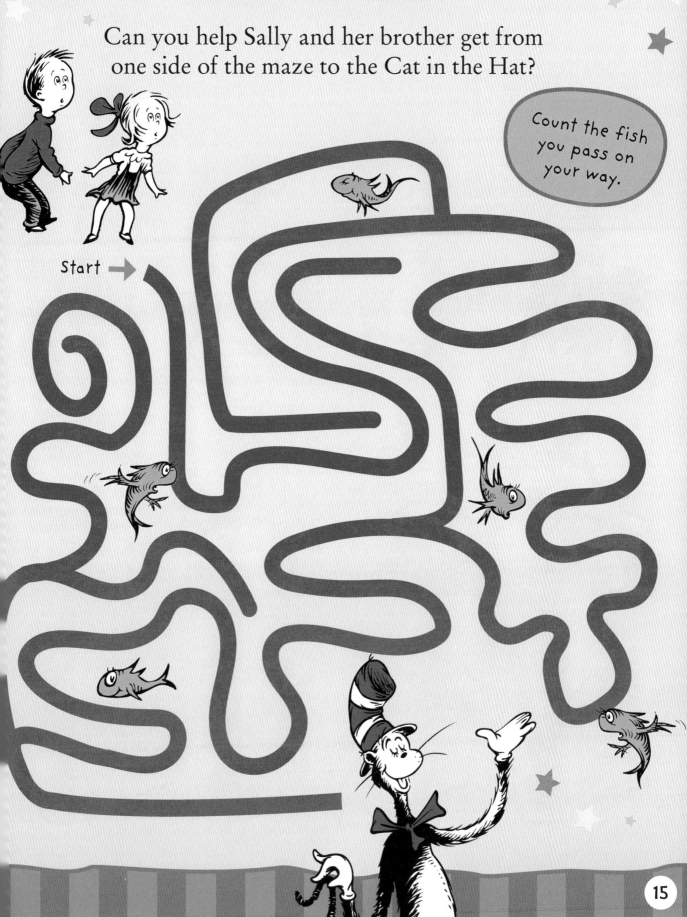

Shadow snap!

Can you find the pictures that match each shadow image?

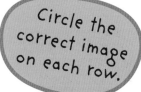

Circle the correct image on each row.

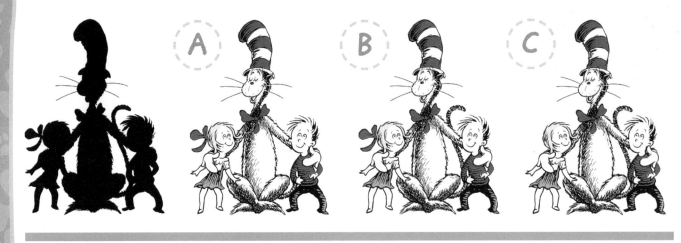

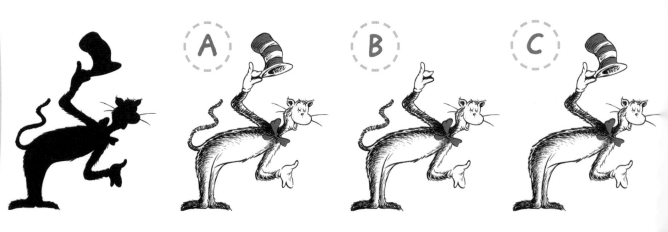

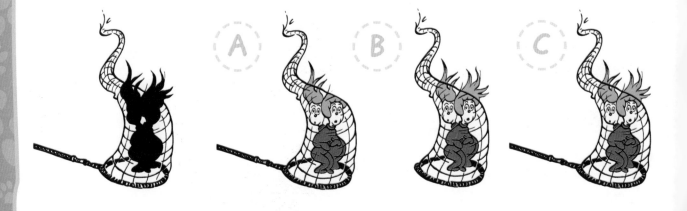

A Hat for the Cat

Can you design a new hat for the Cat? Use your imagination and go wild with your favourite colouring pens and pencils!

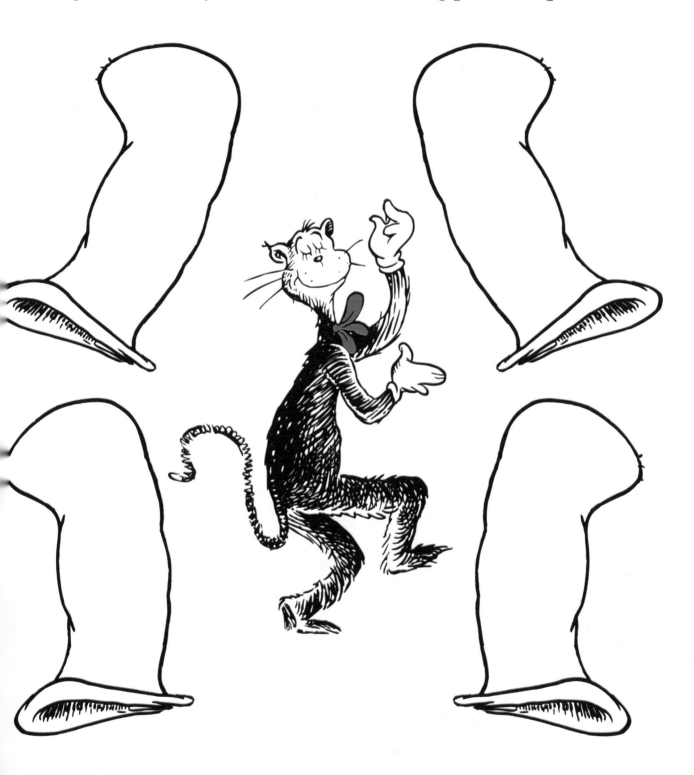

Wonderful wordsearch

Can you find these words in the wordsearch?
They may appear going down or across – so get thinking!

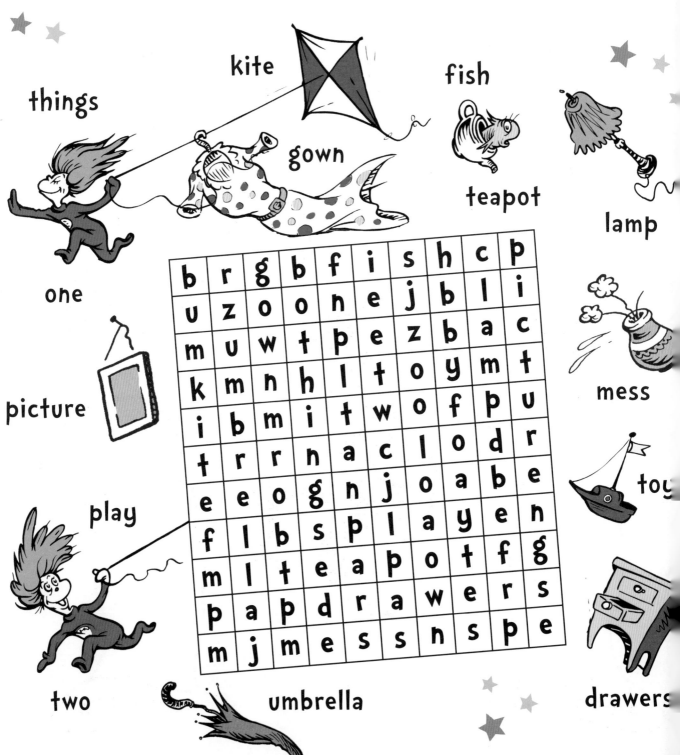

things

kite

fish

gown

teapot

lamp

one

picture

mess

play

toy

two

umbrella

drawers

b	r	g	b	f	i	s	h	c	p
u	z	o	o	n	e	j	b	l	i
m	u	w	t	p	e	z	b	a	c
k	m	n	h	l	t	o	y	m	t
i	b	m	i	t	w	o	f	p	u
t	r	r	n	a	c	l	o	d	r
e	e	o	g	n	j	o	a	b	e
f	l	b	s	p	l	a	y	e	n
m	l	t	e	a	p	o	t	f	g
p	a	p	d	r	a	w	e	r	s
m	j	m	e	s	s	n	s	p	e

An unwanted mess!

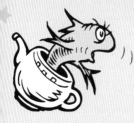

Let's find the matching stickers
for the story below!

"Now look at this house!

Look at this! Look at that!

You sank our toy 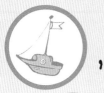,

Sank it deep in the .

You shook up our house

And you bent our new 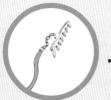.

You SHOULD NOT be here

When our mother is not.

You get out of this house!"

Said the  in the pot.

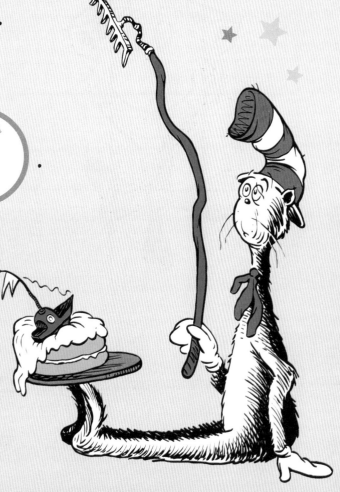

Copy-cat!

Let's copy this image of the Cat in the Hat on to the grid below!

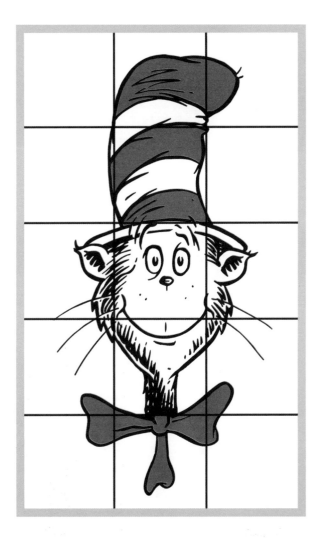

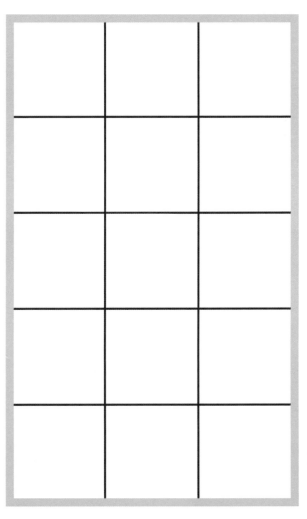

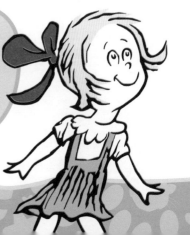

Make sure to use your brightest pens and pencils to colour in the image after!

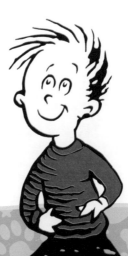

Counting chaos!

How many of each item can you spot in the image below?

Vases ▢ Picture frames ▢ Lampshades ▢ Things ▢

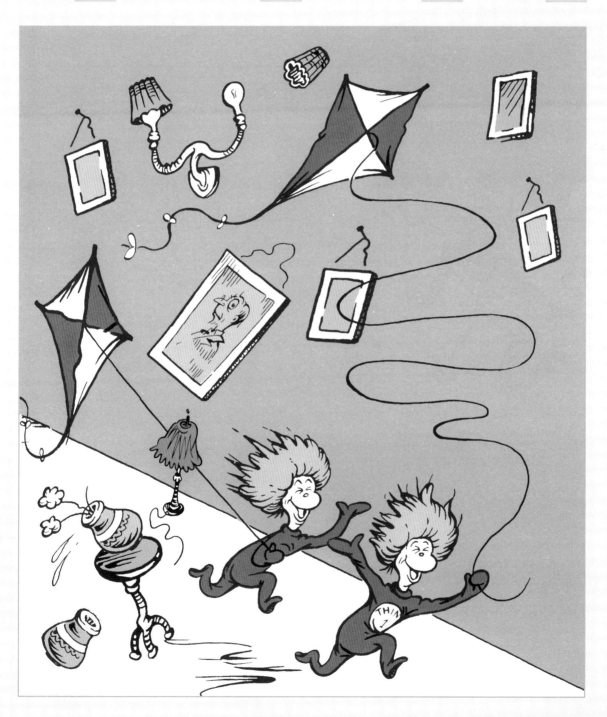

Goodbye, Thing One and Two

It's time for Thing One and Thing Two to return to their box.
Which path leads to this cheeky pair?

Circle the correct number.

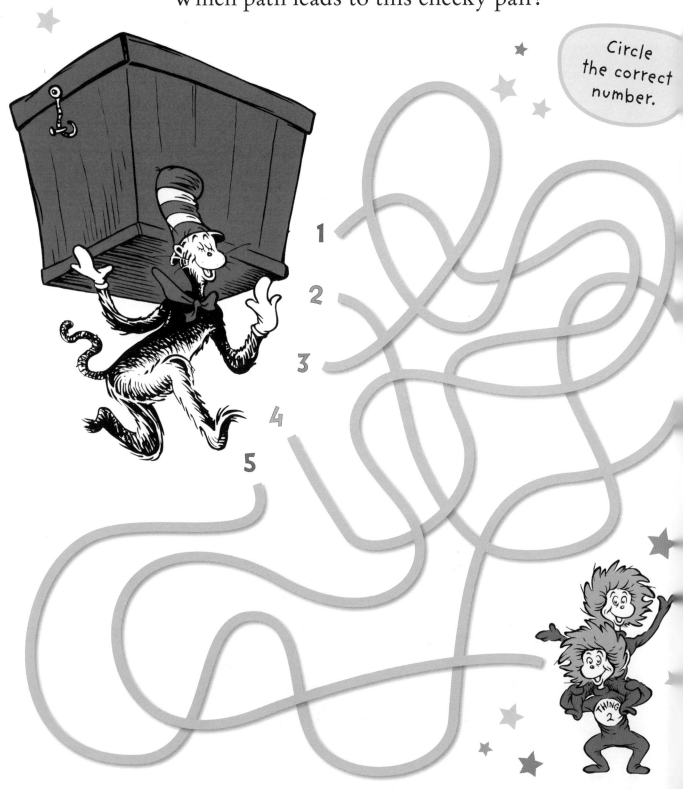

1
2
3
4
5

Detective time!

Decipher the clues below to find Sally and her brother's favourite toy.

Circle the correct item and find the matching sticker.

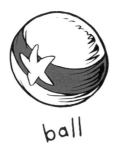
ball

Clue 1. It's red.

Clue 2. You can play with it.

Clue 3. It goes on water.

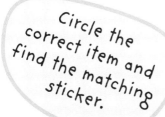
dress

_ _ _ _ _
Write your answer here.

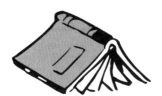
fan

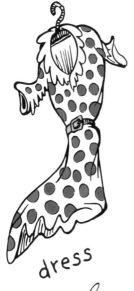
dress

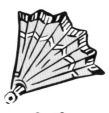
boat

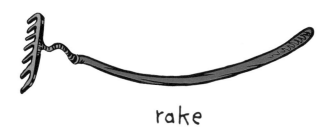
rake

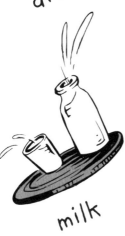
milk

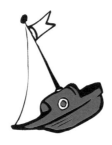

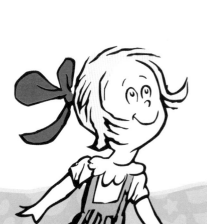

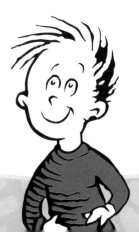

23

Complete the pattern

What comes next in each row?

Find the correct sticker.

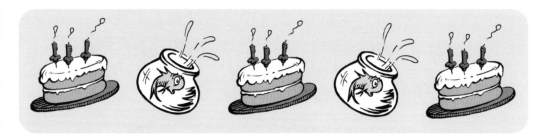

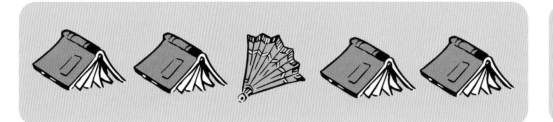

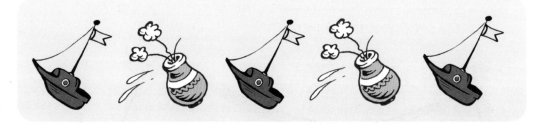

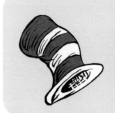   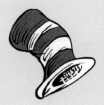 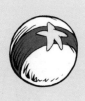

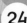

The missing piece

Can you find the right piece to complete the puzzle from the options below?

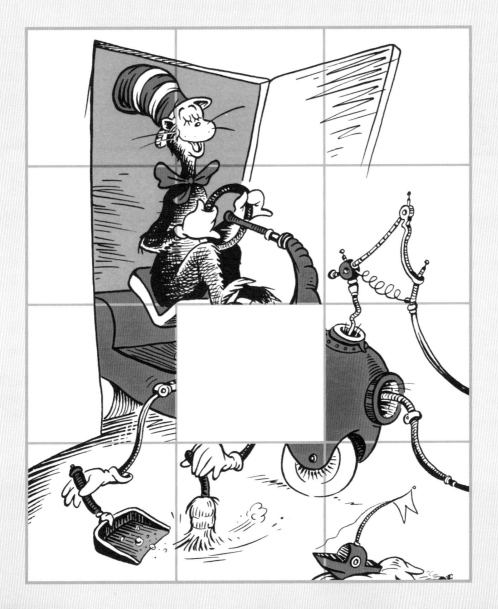

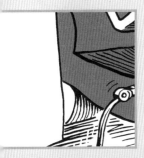
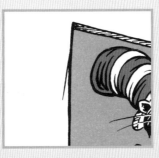
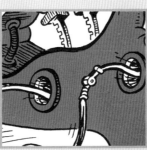

See if you're right by finding the matching sticker!

Matching pairs

Let's help the Cat in the Hat tidy up by sorting the messy things into matching pairs. Draw lines between each pair and then colour in the matching items.

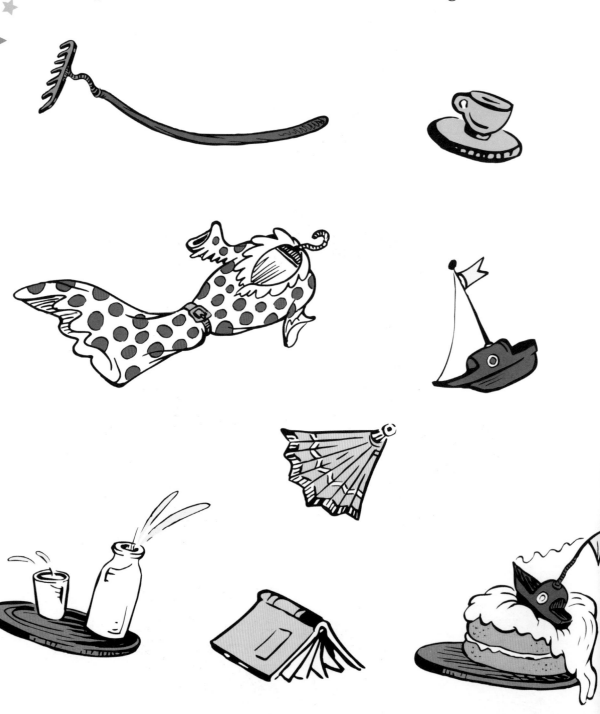

Tick the boxes when you have matched each pair,
but look out – is there one missing?

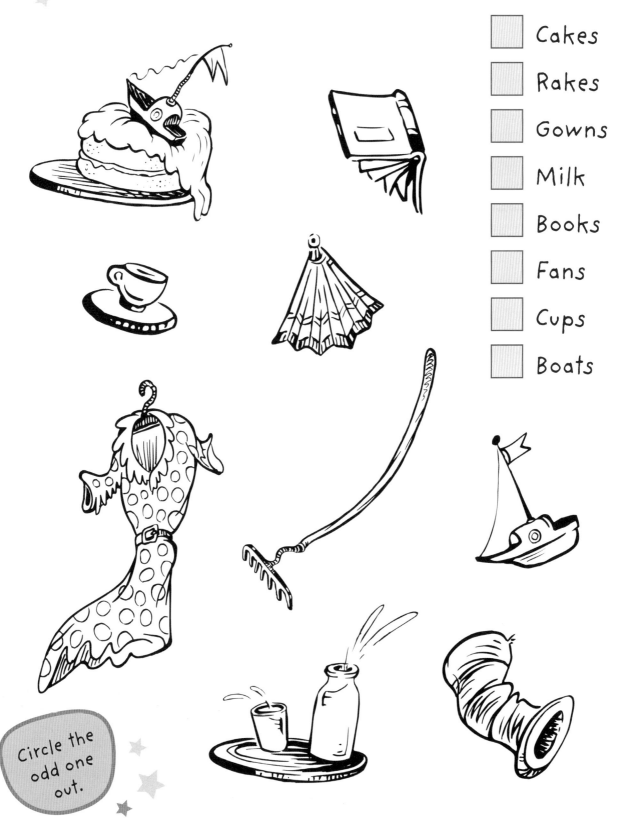

- [ ] Cakes
- [ ] Rakes
- [ ] Gowns
- [ ] Milk
- [ ] Books
- [ ] Fans
- [ ] Cups
- [ ] Boats

Circle the odd one out.

Tidy-up time

Can you find the matching stickers for the text below?

Then we saw him pick up

All the things that were down.

He picked up the 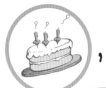,

And the rake, and the 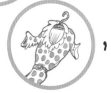,

And the milk, and the strings,

And the , and the dish,

And the fan, and the ,

And the ship,

and the 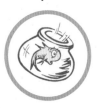.

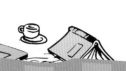
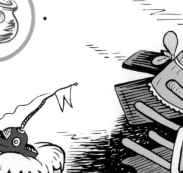
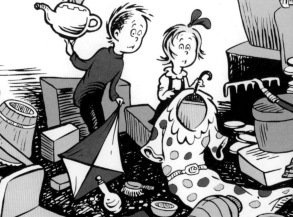

There's the door!

Trace the path to show the Cat in the Hat
the way to the front door.

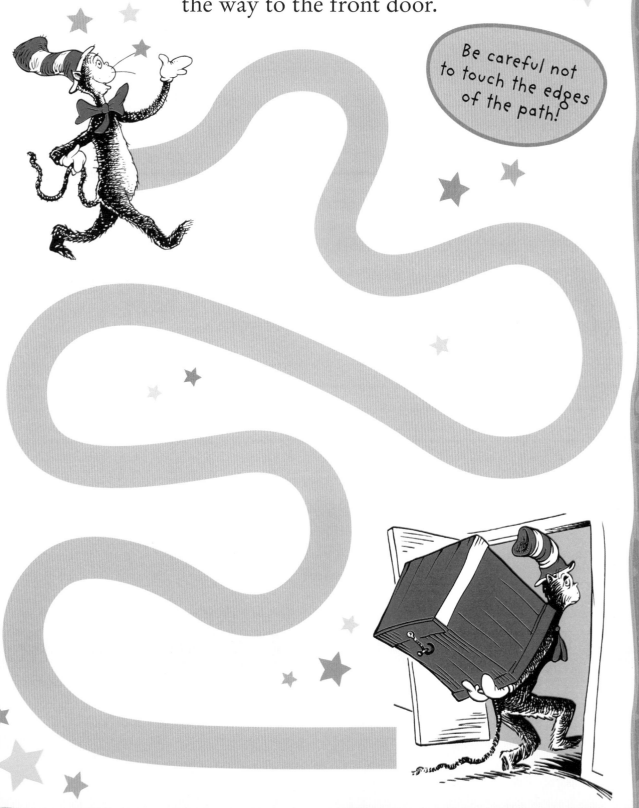

Be careful not
to touch the edges
of the path!

Mother's return

Mother is nearly home! Will Sally and her brother tell her what's happened today?

Can you spot the picture that doesn't match the others? Add a star sticker to the odd one out.

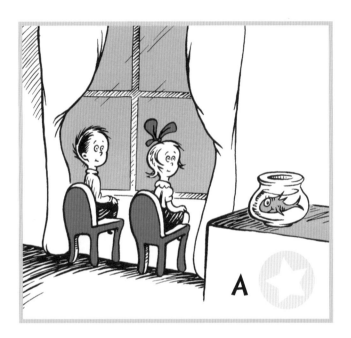

A

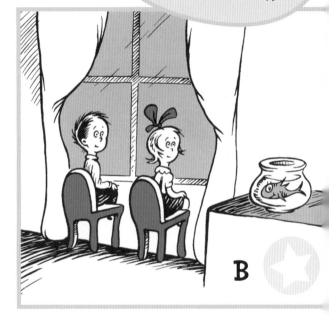

B

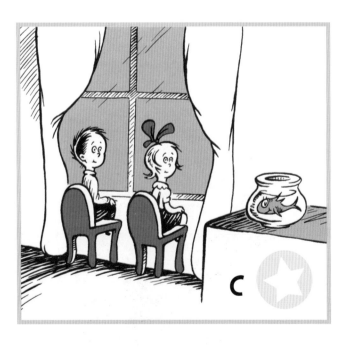

C

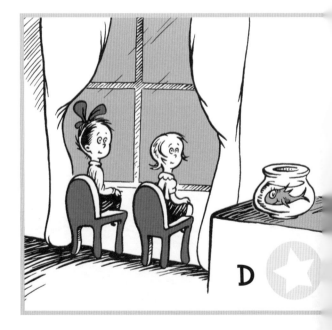

D

Goodbye, Cat in the Hat!

Use your best pens and pencils to add some colour
to the Cat as he goes on his way.

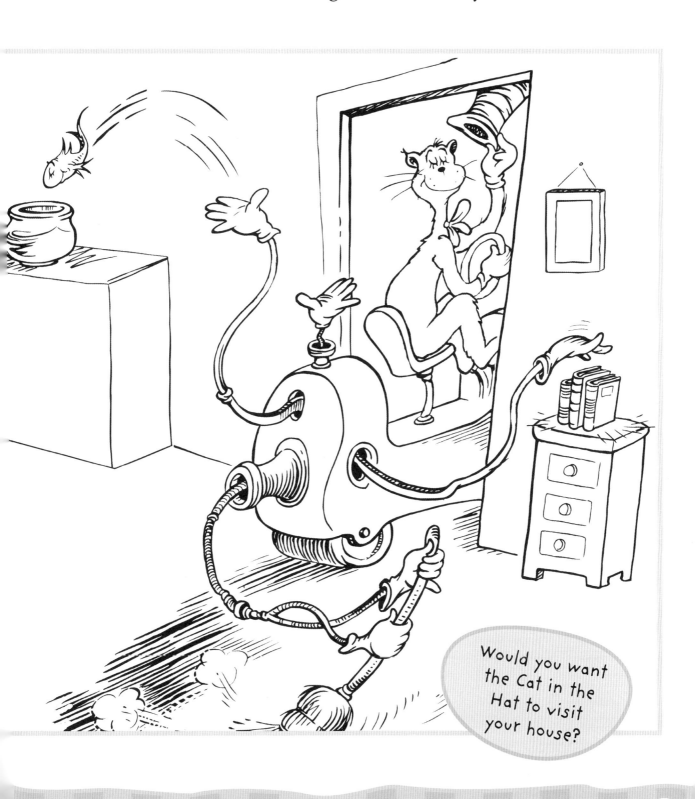

Answers

Page 3

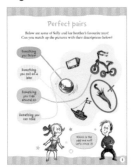

Page 4

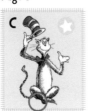

Page 8

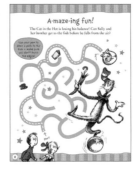

Page 5

Page 7

Page 13

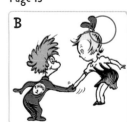

Page 15

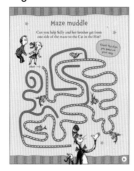

Page 16

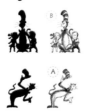

Page 18

Page 21

Page 22

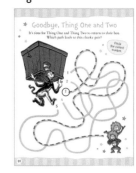

Page 23

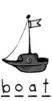

Page 24

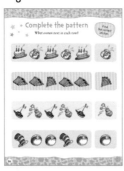

Pages 26–27

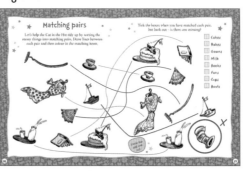

Page 30

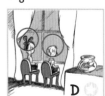

The Cat in the Hat Activity Book
™ & © Dr. Seuss Enterprises, L.P. 1957
All rights reserved

First published in the United Kingdom by HarperCollins *Children's Books* in 2024
HarperCollins *Children's Books* is a division of HarperCollins*Publishers* Ltd
1 London Bridge Street
London SE1 9GF

www.harpercollins.co.uk

HarperCollins*Publishers*
Macken House, 39/40 Mayor Street Upper
Dublin 1, D01 C9W8, Ireland

10 9 8 7 6 5 4 3 2 1

978-0-00-863917-4

Contains copyrighted material from the following publications:
The Cat in the Hat © 1957, 1985 by Dr. Seuss Enterprises, L.P. All rights reserved.
Published by arrangement with Random House Inc., New York, USA
First published in the United Kingdom in 1958

The Cat in the Hat 60th Birthday Edition Sticker Activity Book © 2007, 2017 by Dr. Seuss
Enterprises, L.P. All rights reserved.
Published by arrangement with Random House Inc., New York, USA
First published in the United Kingdom in 2017
The Cat in the Hat 50th Birthday Colouring Activity Book © 2007 by Dr. Seuss Enterprises,
L.P. All rights reserved.
Published by arrangement with Random House Inc., New York, USA
First published in the United Kingdom in 2007

A CIP catalogue record for this title is available from the British Library.

Printed and bound in Poland